Gluten-free Gro

Including snacks, ready-to-go meals, and social situations tips

By : Sarah Shak

Copyrights 2023

No part of the materials available through this book may be sold, adapted, copied, photocopied, reproduced, translated or reduced to any electronic medium or machine-readable form, in whole or in part, without prior written consent of the publisher.

For any query, send an email to:
admin@fodlist.com

Disclaimer

The information contained in this book is for information only, it is not replacing professional consultation about cholesterol, and it is not intended to give any medical advice.

Table of Contents

Introduction : *6*

What this book is exactly about: *9*

Chap 1: *12*

How to enjoy a perfect symptom-free life in every situation *12*

Chap 2: *16*

The 5 stages of your evolution as a gluten-sensitive person: *16*

Chap 3: *18*

Accepting *18*

Chap 4: *21*

Learning *21*

Chap 5: *26*

Adapting *26*

Chap 6: *31*

Communicating : *31*

Chap 7: *35*

Enjoying *35*

Part 2 : *38*

Referential social situations and how to deal with them *38*

Situation 1: *39*

Taking care of a gluten-sensitive child *39*
Situation 2: *48*
Who prepares the food? *48*
Situation 3: *52*
How to enjoy your travel *52*
Situation 4: *57*
Kiss without fear *57*
Situation 5: *60*
Enjoy party time: *60*
Situation 6: *64*
Precautions during a hospital stay *64*
Situation 7: *72*
How to stay safe at work : *72*
Situation 8: *79*
How to do your grocery : *79*
Situation 9: *83*
How to stay safe when using Cosmetics: *83*
Situation 10: *88*
Takeout and delivery *88*
Situation 11: *92*
Sport and outdoors activities *92*
Ready to go gluten-free foods & snacks *95*
Gluten free food & grocery list : *103*

Fish..104
Flour..105
Pasta... 106
Grains & Seeds......................................107
Meat...108
Beans & Nuts 109
Beverages.. 110
Cheese...111
Canned Food................................... 112

Introduction :

In my early thirties, I worked as a construction engineer. I had to travel long distances every day from home to the company, and from the company to the construction sites. My work was physically and emotionally demanding. I started to feel weak, devoid of strength, edgy, my skin has become strangely dry, and I suffered from menstrual irregularities.

I started getting bloating, abdominal pain, joints pain, and hair loss. I thought it was the permanent stress I was exposed to that caused these symptoms as well as the unhealthy food I consumed daily. I thought that it was not necessary to make a medical consultation, and since things did not improve, on the contrary, they became worse:
Inability to go to work for several days, intense abdominal pain, and sometimes sudden and inexplicable dizziness, I finally decided to share my suffering on a Facebook group. People there advised me to consult a gastroenterologist. Which I did! Here is what happened...

My first appointment was relatively short in terms of time. It took about 15 minutes, which I found not enough to fully assess my case. The doctor asked me about my symptoms, my lifestyle, my family's history of diseases, and whether or not I was taking any kind of medication. Finally, the doctor asked me to do some blood tests and to go dairy-free and gluten-free until I receive my test results.

Some days after that, the doctor confirmed that I was gluten-intolerant. At the beginning, I was confused. I didn't know if I should be happy to learn that I didn't have a condition that would jeopardize my health, or do I have to worry because now I have to reconsider my entire lifestyle that relies on fast-food, prepared meals, snacks, and quick fixes in general?! I was disturbed to realize that there is no medicine or magic pill that will heal me overnight. I learned that if I want to live a normal life without symptoms, I have to make some major changes to my whole lifestyle, especially my diet.
I understood that I had to give up on fast-food, avoid gluten-rich alimentation, and pay attention to my symptoms.

Until now I was a distracted woman. My time was shared between work and family, and I completely forgot to take care of myself.

During the first weeks after the doctor's visit, I was looking at my gluten intolerance as a curse that would haunt me and ruin my life. However, I now feel blessed.

I realized that it has allowed me to reconnect with myself, meet new great people from different ethnicities, and have access to an energy and self-fulfillment I had never experienced before.

Being gluten-free has completely changed my whole life for the better. I feel healthier, happier, and more confident. I decided to write this book because I truly believe in the power of sharing my experience to help people whether they suffer from celiac, or they have non-celiac gluten sensitivity.

Through this book, I aim to provide guidance, inspiration, and practical advice to help people who are navigating the complexities of managing their dietary needs and lifestyle requirements.

The encouragement and positive feedback I have received from a bunch of friends, colleagues, and other people who have benefited from my experience has strengthened my determination to share it with a wider audience. I hope what you will read and learn in this book will serve you in your life. I hope it will turn your gluten intolerance into a blessed experience as it was for me.

Sarah

What this book is exactly about:

I wrote this book for the sole reason to help you with your daily life!

This book will be your survival guide to almost every situation you face on a daily basis. When I was diagnosed with gluten intolerance, all I could find were books, videos, and articles that explain the mechanism behind gluten sensitivity, gluten-free cookbooks, and some general guidelines like avoiding food that contains wheat, watching out for cross-contamination, etc...but nothing else!

I am a human being, a wife, and a mom. I have a social life. I go to work, I go to the grocery, I meet people, I invite people to my house and I get invited to their houses. I needed someone or at least a guide that will point out to me the things I should pay attention to in these situations. I needed to know what I should do to protect myself, and how to live normally without getting sick...but I couldn't find anything like that. This book is an attempt to fill this void in the gluten intolerance and celiac books library.

You will not find medical terms in this book, and this book is not the right one if you want to learn how gluten sensitivity works. There are videos, articles, and other books that cover this subject perfectly.

Are you invited to a wedding party, and would like to know what to do to enjoy your time without getting sick? Do you want to travel and enjoy your trip without experiencing any symptoms? Are you forced to stay in the hospital for some days, and want to know what preparations you need to make?... This book will give you the exact and right answers to these questions.

You will find guidelines, tips, and strategies drawn from my personal experience and from other people's experiences like you. These guidelines will literally save you countless times in countless situations. But that's not all...

This book also will guide you through your gluten-free journey in every aspect of your life. You will discover that gluten intolerance whether it is celiac or non-celiac shouldn't be a curse. In fact, you will learn how to enjoy it and help other gluten-intolerant people too. The first chapters of this book cover this subject in a structural and simple way. I invite you to read them thoroughly as they lay down the foundation for the upcoming ones.

Basically, this book is made up of three main parts:

Part one: from chapter 1 to chapter 7. In this part, you will learn how to deal with gluten intolerance, and how to enjoy your life as a gluten intolerant.

Part 2: In this part, you will learn what exactly to do in different life situations to protect yourself from getting contaminated, enjoy social life, and food.

Part 3: A comprehensive list of real gluten-free foods you can eat or use as ingredients for cooking.

Soon, this book will be your favorite supportive friend on your journey!

Chap 1:

How to enjoy a perfect symptom-free life in every situation

Gluten patients fall into the trap of identifying themselves with this condition. When I meet gluten-sensitive people for the first time and they want to introduce themselves, 90% of them state their names, and then they say "I am gluten intolerant" even though I didn't ask if they have any health condition or not. Gluten sensitivity is a special physiological condition and should remain so. It should not be part of your identity or your personality.

If there is an accurate name other than gluten sensitivity whether caused by celiac or not, it would be the contamination/starvation game. Managing gluten sensitivity boils down to two things: starvation and contamination. If you can control those two facts, you have won over gluten intolerance. Another aspect that bothers me is associating gluten intolerance with socialization. Gluten patients tend to think that their condition will limit their interaction with others. They believe in that and behave accordingly. As a result of this misconception, they finish imprisoned in the "Gluten

Box", which is a description of isolation and low self-confidence in some gluten-sensitivity patients.

So let me say it again, gluten intolerance has nothing to do with socialization. It is a game of contamination and starvation. You can perfectly socialize whenever and wherever the opportunity presents itself to you, without refraining from enjoying social interaction with others.

If you are looking for a simple, practical, and extremely efficient way to have a perfect symptom-free life on a daily basis, then here it is:
The gluten-intolerance ecosystem is made up of three components:

1. **You**
2. **The environment**
3. **The time**

If I could live for years without gluten sensitivity symptoms, and almost heal myself, it is because I ask myself three questions related to the above components:

Q1: Is it easy to get gluten-free food in that environment in case of emergency?
Q2: For how long I will stay in that environment?

Q3: What do I have to do in order to stay safe in that environment?

Let me give you an example. Imagine you were invited to a wedding party. Then in order to enjoy your time, socialize, and do what a normal person would do at a wedding party, you should answer these three questions: Is it easy to get gluten-free food at that wedding party? The answer will be "Yes" most likely if there are fruits and vegetables there, or if the party is held in a city where you can get gluten-free food delivered to you in case of emergency.

The next question is: how long will you stay at that party? Less than 3 hours or more than that?
And lastly, what you should do to protect yourself, and enjoy your time?
As a general rule of thumb, if I have to stay in a place for three hours and more, I either cook my food and take it with me or order it using food delivery apps. By contrast, if I stay less than three hours, I eat very well before going out, so my mind will not get busy with food ideas. And thus, I will have time to enjoy and socialize.

Since the first time I figured out these guidelines and started applying them for years now, I have never gotten sick. These guidelines have served me to separate myself as a human being from my condition as gluten intolerant, and have allowed me to perfectly control the contamination/starvation dilemma.

I have also developed customized measures for each situation and each environment. The next pages of this book are all about that. Use them, improve them, modify them to suit you, and add yours as you become more experienced and more familiar with them.

I strongly encourage you to share your tips with others, and I will be extremely happy if you share them with me so they will be my inspiration to make the next edition of this book even better, and more useful.

Chap 2:

The 5 stages of your evolution as a gluten-sensitive person:

The 5 stages of your evolution as a gluten-sensitive person:

As I said in the intro of this book, I will not dive into the medical side of gluten sensitivity. Instead, I will focus only and mainly on what will serve you in your daily life. So based on this, let's talk about the six stages of your evolution as a gluten-sensitive person. I will briefly state each one of them in this chapter, and I will expand on each separately in the next chapter.

Each gluten person will navigate (probably) 5 states in his life while dealing with gluten intolerance. These states are:

1. **Accepting**
2. **Learning**
3. **Adapting**
4. **Communicating**
5. **Enjoying**

These stages are like the steps of stairs, which mean you will not be able to move to a stage without being in the stage before it. This also means that when you master a stage, you will move automatically to the next stage. The first step is the "Accepting" stage, and the last one is the "Contributing" stage.

The majority of gluten-sensitivity patients are somewhere between stage 1 and stage 4. These are the people who are trying to cope with their gluten intolerance. They have enough knowledge and experience to eat the right food, avoid contamination sources, and communicate their dietary needs whenever necessary. However, they hadn't yet reached the stage of enjoying the gluten-free lifestyle and its benefits. I was one of them, and there is a good chance you are one of them too. However, I learned how to love my new life, and actually benefit from it physically, emotionally, and financially. I will show you how to achieve similar (or even better) results in the coming pages. So stay with me.

Now let's go through the first stage:

Accepting.

Chap 3:

Accepting

Accepting to be a gluten-intolerant person, to be part of this group with specific dietary needs, was a major step for me, as it will be for you as well!

By accepting your gluten intolerance, you communicate a clear and precise message to your body and especially to your mind. This message is: "Everything will be fine; we will find a solution to this situation". In other words, you choose to take an active role in your intolerance and take charge of yourself. This opens the door to understanding your body's unique needs, and discovering how to support your health and well-being.

Additionally, acceptance releases you from the emotional turmoil that comes with struggling with your condition. Instead, acceptance nurtures compassion for yourself, which promotes emotional well-being and allows you to cultivate a positive relationship with yourself and your body.

During the research phase to write this book, and to understand in a more concrete way the enormous positive impact that acceptance had on my emotional and bodily state, I came across the research work done on this subject by Dr. Jazaieri et al in 2013. In this study, participants were trained to embrace the culture of acceptance and compassion.

Researchers found that engaging in acceptance practices significantly increased the activity in areas of the brain associated with emotional regulation, and decreased the activity in areas related to stress and anxiety. These changes elicited a sense of emotional well-being in the participants.

The study highlights the power of acceptance to influence chemicals in the brain and nervous system.

Acceptance-based practices promote a state of relaxation, reduce stress hormone levels, and increase the release of feel-good neurotransmitters like serotonin and endorphins. These changes contribute to improved mood, reduced anxiety, and overall mental well-being.

Stress is a major catalyst for gluten intolerance symptoms. If you are stressed, your sensitivity to gluten increases, your digestive system works even worse, and your body releases more of the hormone cortisol, thus aggravating the inflammation caused by gluten intolerance, which further intensifies your symptoms and makes them more frequent.

Acceptance also opens the door to seeking support and connecting with others like you. It allows you to seek out and exchange advice, resources, and experiences with others – like what I am trying to do with you through this book - and, improve your ability to manage your gluten intolerance with confidence and resilience.

Remember, acceptance does not mean resignation or quitting. It is a powerful choice for embracing your reality and making the most of it. By accepting your gluten intolerance, you give yourself the means to live a fulfilled, healthy, and above all stress-free life.

Chap 4:

Learning

As a beginner in the world of gluten sensitivity, the major question you will face is not: "What to learn?", but "How to learn what to learn?". Let me explain...

When I was diagnosed with gluten intolerance, I had no idea about the nature of this condition. I had no idea how it is triggered, how it is healed, what medicines or remedies are available for it,...I used to go online, type in some general keywords like "Gluten intolerance" in the search bar, and click on the search results one by one.

It took me valuable time to learn about contamination, reading food labels, gluten-free foods, available gluten-free options...etc. Meanwhile, I was suffering from gluten symptoms caused by consuming either contaminated or the wrong food. If just someone took 15 minutes to teach me what I should learn, it would spare me days of stress, and countless sleepless nights.

I will spare you the headache of trying to figure out what to know to avoid health problems caused by the gluten sensitivity whether it is celiac or non-celiac. I will give in a logical order what you should learn by the end of this chapter, which will make your learning curve considerably shorter . However, I would like to highlight an important fact in this regard.

No one on this planet, even the most experienced and skilled gluten-sensitivity doctor will be able to teach you like your own body. Each one of us is unique, and so is each one's reaction to gluten.

I know people who get sick just by touching gluten-containing things with their naked hands, others get sick just by inhaling, and others consume some gluten-containing foods without triggering any symptoms! Yes, when you apply the guidelines in this book you will rarely get sick, but when you do, listen to what your body has to tell you, write down your symptoms, write down what you ate in the last 48 hours, and when you do that, you will start noticing patterns about foods, situations, and things that irritate your body. When you do that, you hit a home run! You will be able to avoid them and have more control over your life.

In addition to what has been said, I would like to highlight the importance of learning in small steps. Whenever people ask me about my gluten-free book recommendations, my answer surprises them! I have never recommended cookbooks, or books that explain and expand on gluten intolerance. Before I wrote this book, I only recommend one book to every gluten-intolerance beginner. This book is the "Compound Effect".

New gluten intolerance patients generally get overwhelmed, and confused when they look at the amount of information they should know, which makes them stressed. I recommend "the Compound Effect" because it teaches how to learn anything in life and master it in a way that almost guarantees the end goal without stress. Now I add the book you are reading right now to the list of my recommendation.

If you are reading this book on a screen, I would suggest you get the paperback copy because you will need to take notes, add your remarks, and your own tips.

I have designed a 7-day learning plan to put you on a fast track. This plan is the result of my experience as a gluten-intolerant person, and the feedback I get from other patients.

This plan as well as all the tips in this book are flexible, meaning you can adapt them to your specific needs. If something does not resonate with your lifestyle, it is perfectly fine to modify it to suit you, or you can ignore it if you choose to. My aim is to keep you connected with your body while providing you with the best material to help you with your gluten intolerance.

Here is the 7-day learning plan:

Day 1: Get a Basic Understanding of Gluten Intolerance

- Learn what it is and how it affects the body. (10 minutes)
- Read about common symptoms and signs of gluten intolerance to help you identify them in your own experience. (15 min)

Day 2: Introduction to Gluten-Containing Foods

- Read about common sources of gluten, such as wheat, barley, and rye (20 min)
- Learn to read food labels and identify ingredients that may contain gluten. (20 min)

Day 3: Introduction to Gluten-Free Foods

- Read about gluten-free alternatives and safe food options for your diet. (30-40 min)

- Explore the list in the appendix of this book of naturally gluten-free foods like fruits, vegetables, meats, and dairy products (20 min)

Day 4: Cross-contamination

- Read about cross-contamination and its causes. (20-30 min)

Day 5: Gluten-Free Cooking and Baking

- Discover gluten-free recipes and cooking techniques that can help you enjoy a diverse range of meals. (40-50 min)

Day 6: Eating Out and Social Settings

- Read part 2 chapters your awareness about tips and strategies in social situations

Day 7: Support

- Join online communities of gluten-intolerant people, and be active there. I recommend Facebook groups.

Chap 5:

Adapting

Learning and adapting go hand in hand. The more you learn, the easier it will be for you to adapt to the gluten-intolerant lifestyle. When my doctor announced to me that I was gluten intolerant, the first thought that hit my mind was "Adaptation".

If you think about it, you will realize that all gluten-related books, articles, videos, shows, and the whole gluten-free industry have a core mission: Helping you to adapt, and thanks to this, it has become incredibly easier now than it was 5 years ago.

I am not talking only about food and dietary needs. The adaptation is more inclusive than that. It covers your social life, your working life, and even your intimate moments with your partner. I tried to cover these aspects in this book, and I believe you will find this work extremely helpful. But as I said before, you are special, your conditions are special, and your body is special. You are the one in control, so keep learning, and keep adapting.

As a gluten-intolerant, you will deal with two environments: an internal and an external environment. The internal one is made up of people you live with and share food with. These people may be your parents, your husband, your wife, a partner you are living with, etc...By contrast, the external environment is anyone else: friends, colleagues, people you meet at a party, etc...

The internal environment is the most challenging to adapt to, but at the same time has the most significant impact on your life either positively or negatively as a gluten-intolerant person. Fortunately, the majority of gluten patients I have met are living in a supportive internal environment that empowers them, but there are other cases where it is completely the opposite that is happening.

I insist on building a supportive internal environment as it will be your best ally when you deal with the external one, and that won't be possible in the lack of proper communication, and compassion. I will never forget the face of that woman who visited me in my office 6 months ago. Let's call her Natasha to protect her privacy.

From the second our eyes met, I could feel she was suffering, and I was right! She sat down on the chair in front of me, and the first thing she did was crying. I asked her what was going on, and she replied with a shaking voice and tears in her eyes that her husband was hurting her! She told me they were married for 15 years, they have 3 wonderful children and everything was going well until she was diagnosed with celiac 1 year ago. She described several situations where her husband got angry about food, and didn't hold back from manifesting his anger through hurting words and actions, but what really pushed her to the edge, and brought her to my office is when he said (I report exactly her own words): "If I could know you would get this F* celiac or whatever it is called, I would think twice before marrying you!"

Natasha's case was an extreme one, and it is very rare. We invited the husband to explain to him everything he needs to know about his wife's condition. We also involved a social assistant and a therapist to save the couple's marriage, and they are doing well together right now. However, when I spoke to the husband, I could understand that the wife didn't take the time to explain to her husband the implications of her condition and the risk involved if she consumes the wrong food, which was a major mistake from her side.

When you have a supportive internal environment, like the people you live with in your house, they will be happy to adjust a little bit their eating habits to match your gluten-free eating mode. You will be as result of that less stressed about food, you will be able to enjoy your meals, you will have the time, the mood, and the motivation to take care of yourself, to focus on your goals, and to prepare for social situations that take place in external environments. Even if you get contaminated by mistake or ignorance, your internal environment will support you, and help you to recover.

When you have a supportive internal environment where you can eat safely, then why should you care if you can't have food at the neighborhood children's birthday parties? Why you should care if you can't find proper food at your friends' wedding parties? Just eat before leaving your house, or prepare the food and take it with you. I invite you to read the chapters of the part 2 of this book to gain more insight into how to run a safe internal environment, and how to adapt it to your needs.

As gluten intolerant, you should have a safe zone, you can also name it your private zone where you can prepare or keep your gluten-free food and snacks. This zone could be as simple as a dedicated place in your kitchen for cooking gluten-free food, a small area in the fridge where you keep your food fresh and protected from contamination, or just a drawer where you store your gluten-free snacks. Having this area at home will provide you with a sense of security, control, and serve as a last-resort food source in emergency cases.

Last but not least, you must keep a personal notebook for your gluten intolerance. This notebook will be the most powerful tool to help you adapt, adjust your lifestyle, and even heal yourself! When symptoms appear, check what you have done and eaten in the last 48h. Do you feel tired? Then check your last 48 h? You can't focus today? Then look at the last 48h, and so on...

I don't recommend at all using phone apps to take notes, because each time you open your phone there is a huge chance you will get distracted by notifications, messages, and so on...your will power will not help you stay focused when taking notes, because Silicon Valley's engineers are working hard to the bone to grab your attention, and you will not escape them once you open up your phone. I refer you to the book "Stolen Focus" if you want to learn what these people are doing to keep you attached to your smart device. I also don't recommend using phone apps because they don't offer the same freedom and speed of writing as pen and paper.

Chap 6:
Communicating :

There is a direct correlation between proper communication, and being in good physical and emotional health as a gluten-intolerant. The basic role of communication is to express thoughts and feelings, and as a gluten-intolerant, you should do that as a kid would do it!

If something has the potential to harm your health, don't hold back. Say it, express it, and don't be ashamed of it! Your health is more important than anything else, and it should be your first priority!

As a society and humans that live together and interact in civilized cities, we have established social rules by which we abide by choice, like avoiding rude words and actions, being polite with others, etc...These rules are general, but at the same time remain flexible depending on each one's situation.

One of my close friends was once invited to dinner. She has celiac, and she asked me if it was rude to tell the host about her dietary needs. I told her that's not rude at all, and she must communicate her food restrictions to the host. I explained to her that what is really inappropriate, and unpardonable is to let the host spend time, money, and energy on preparing food that she won't eat. By contrast, she will inspire respect if she explains her condition, and shows her concern about the effort the host would make to prepare that food. If you were the host, what would you think of her?

There are two types of communication: verbal and non-verbal. Verbal is when you use words to express your thoughts, and non-verbal is when you use something else other than words. As gluten-intolerant, both types will serve you in different ways depending on the situation. Some examples of non-verbal communication include: Wearing bracelets, necklaces, T-shirts, hats...that express you are a gluten-intolerant person. This also includes the stickers you put on your water bottle, or on your bento box to prevent others from touching them, and causing food contamination.

The most obvious case when verbal and non-verbal communication are equally important is when you have a gluten-intolerant child. In this case, your primary concern is to keep him safe while being in the external environment, and this couldn't be possible without talking to people who have direct interaction with him, making him wear bracelets, accessories, or anything else that will alert adults and prevent them from giving him bad food. **Please refer to the "Taking Care Of A Gluten-Free Child" chapter,** which explains and expands on this case.

The people you are living with should also be at the top of your communication list. A gluten-free lifestyle is challenging at the beginning. It involves making adjustments to your dietary habits as well as to those of people who live with you in the same house.

Talking about your needs clearly, asking for support openly, and answering their questions without shame is the most effective way I know to keep the peace and warmth between you and them. They have the right to ask questions about your gluten intolerance, and they have the right to express their concerns when you separate your food from theirs, so don't be bothered, consider it as a learning period for them to learn how to better support you, it will pass, be open-minded and express your gratitude because you live with such wonderful people who care about you!

Here are some actionable communication tips I recommend:

Educate others: Provide basic information about your gluten intolerance and what the consumption of the wrong food may cause you.

Use assertive language: Use assertive statements to communicate your dietary requirements. For example, say, "I must avoid gluten due to celiac disease" rather than apologizing or downplaying your needs.

Communicate with confidence: Project confidence when discussing your dietary needs. This will help others understand the importance of gluten-free diets and reduce misunderstandings.

Express gratitude: Show appreciation to those who accommodate your dietary needs. Thank restaurant staff, friends, or family members who make an effort to provide gluten-free options. This positive reinforcement encourages continued support and understanding.

Chap 7:
Enjoying

There are three dimensions that should be considered if you would like to enjoy a gluten-free lifestyle:

1. Your relationship with yourself
2. Your relationship with food
3. Your relationship with the external world

In other words, having a healthy link with yourself, food, and society will propel you from survival mode into enjoyment mode as a gluten intolerant. Through the chapters: Accepting, Learning, Adapting, and Communicating, I covered the guidelines that will help you achieve that successfully. However, in this chapter, I would like to emphasize the importance of another ingredient that will make your life perfect as a gluten intolerant, and this ingredient is: Contribution.

As I said before, the problem with the material available for gluten-intolerant persons is limited to cookbooks and material that explains the mechanisms behind the gluten intolerance condition. This kind of material surely is useful, but it serves inherently only in survival mode, in other words, it helps only to cope with this condition, but not to control it and enjoy it! I was like that at the beginning with my gluten intolerance, and this is why I wrote this book for you! I want to pull you out from survival mode to enjoying mode. This book is my contribution, it is my giving back, and I have enjoyed writing each word of it.

The beauty of contribution is that you will always benefit from something bigger and more beautiful in return. I once heard someone say this phrase: "If you help enough people get what they want, you will get everything you want". Speaking of myself, I have met wonderful people at the association I work with. These people had a profound impact on my personal and financial life that I couldn't imagine in my wildest dreams. This book also generates royalties that are intended to support other people financially (by the way, thank you for purchasing it! I really appreciate it!). Also helping others stand above their daily struggles as gluten intolerant gives deep meaning to my life, and has become an essence of internal joy and peace that nothing in this world can shake it!

As a gluten intolerant, you are the best-qualified person to help other folks like you. You feel what they feel. They face the same challenges, obstacles, and maybe similar social situations, so why not extend a helping hand to them? This is also a path for you to acquire more knowledge and experience that will help you get better with your own gluten-free life.

Contribute from your standpoint to make life easier and better for other gluten-intolerant buddies. Your contribution could be as small as giving a piece of advice in a Facebook group. It could also be sharing a recipe you have tested and enjoyed, writing a blog post, or recommending this book or any other material. Don't underestimate the value of your contribution. You never know who will benefit from it!

Another reason I urge you to contribute is that the gluten-intolerant community needs you. The gluten-free market is extremely profitable and expanding day in and day out. However, until the time of writing this book, gluten regulation in the US, UK, and other countries is very loose. Getting the gluten-free label is relatively simple, and companies abusing this regulation are mushrooming at the speed of light. That explains why people get gluten reaction attacks when they consume some gluten-free labeled food. So in order to stop this flood, we need to build a strong community, and that will not be possible without your contribution.

Part 2 :

Referential social situations and how to deal with them

Situation 1:

Taking care of a gluten-sensitive child

Being sensitive to gluten as an adult is challenging if you lack proper guidance and people to support you throughout your learning phase. However, living with a gluten-sensitive kid is a completely different story.

This chapter was the first I thought about before writing a single word in this book, and that's because when gluten intolerance hits kids, it becomes a social and psychological matter more than it is a health matter. I have seen poor parents experiencing difficult moments with their kids because their relatives, friends, or even strangers they met for the first time make a comment, act, or behave in a way that hurts their kids. In the association I work with, I have daily contact and close interaction with mothers and fathers that are trying to make their way through this. They have to wear a psychologist hat to answer their kids' questions about their gluten intolerance, and why they couldn't eat whatever they wanted or behave normally - like other kids of their age.

Not long ago, before I resolved to write this book, I sat down with these parents and asked them one single question: "What is your biggest challenge in managing your kid's gluten intolerance?" I got three main answers. Here are the statistics:

- 40% Said: Family and relatives don't respect their kid's dietary needs or don't understand them.

- 30% Said: Food served in schools is gluten-contaminated

- 30%: Different reasons

As you can see from the previous figures, family plays a big part in the life of a gluten-intolerant kid. Let me tell you a real-life story to illustrate this...

I was sitting at my desk one evening. I remember it was Mai, it was 11 o'clock morning (if I remember well), and I heard someone knocking on the door and asking permission to come in. She was Marianne, a young lady with blond hair, and blue beautiful eyes. After greetings, she started to tell me her story about her gluten-intolerant daughter, and how she is badly affected by her family. I was startled listening to what she was saying, and I was wondering how she could manage this enormous amount of stress given her young age. She was 26 years old. She said:

" My daughter was diagnosed with celiac just over a year ago when she was 5 years old. We made the decision to go gluten-free to make it easier for her, but my husband's family members just don't understand her dietary needs. Every time she visits her grandparents, she gets really sick because of the food they give her. I remember that night when she was at her uncle's house to attend his son's birthday with other kids in the family. They have sworn they would make special treats for her, but they didn't keep their promise. When she came back home, she was screaming out of pain. We took her to the hospital, and she stayed there the whole night! I was angry and upset! Her father was extremely panicking. He grabbed his phone, called his brother, and almost fought over the line! We didn't exchange words with her uncle's family since then. My husband's parents blame him for being overprotective of his daughter and tell him to let her face the difficulties of life so she can learn and grow, but he really doesn't care. We have agreed that what counts is our daughter's health. We will protect her whatever it takes until she reaches the age to able to take care of herself.

We become strict with anyone who doesn't respect our daughter's boundaries. We communicate clearly, and bluntly her needs to all family members, and to anyone wanting her as a host at his kid's birthday party. We don't give a second chance to anyone who breaks these rules. We are clear: "If she gets sick while you are with her, you will never see her again!" We still see some kind of resistance, and misbehavior - Especially in the school- from people thinking gluten is not a matter to worry about, but, we take this as proof that we are - As parents- doing our best to protect our sweety"

End of Marianne's words.

I am not in a position to judge Marianne's behavior or give her advice about how to build better relationships with her husband's family. However, I appreciate her advocacy for her daughter and her commitment to protecting her. Parents are often faced with two options:

Option 1: Being protective, which means - sometimes - being harsh with people that harm their children

Option 2: Being polite with people around them, and trying to educate them about their children's condition.

It is clear that Marianne has chosen the first option, and you may too, but let's be honest, if your kid gets sick each time he is at your relative's house, then, what's the point in trying to educate him?

From what I could see, and contrary to the folks you hang with online, the majority of people around you in real life don't know anything about celiac and gluten sensitivity. Even the ones you think are aware see gluten intolerance as a diet you choose to follow (like the keto diet for example), not an imposed condition that could make you sick if you eat the wrong food. They make their own assumptions and conclusions, and let you pay the consequences with your health or your kid's health. From time to time I get messages like this: " My kid got contaminated because his grandparents thought if you cook the food long enough, the gluten in the food will disappear"!

If you need to set boundaries and be harsh to protect your kid, then no one has the right to blame you, because no one will be with you in the hospital, when you are trying to explain to your kid why this happened to him, or why he couldn't eat like other kids. It's your duty as a parent, and believe me, you will be grateful when you look back at it years from now.

Taking care of the psychological needs of your kid is as crucial as taking care of his dietary needs. Remember, your kid is a "Kid", he needs to play, hang out with other kids, and socialize with others. Don't mistake protection for imprisonment. Studies have shown that people that have specific dietary needs are 3X times more exposed to eating disorders than normal people.

The ADHD (Attention-Deficit/Hyperactivity Disorder) is a condition affecting more and more kids globally, especially in the United States, and the United Kingdom. It is characterized by symptoms of inattention, hyperactivity, and impulsivity. Kids with ADHD may have difficulties with sustaining attention, organizing tasks, maintaining focus, and controlling impulsive behaviors that can affect their learning abilities.

Johann Hari has written a great book called "Stolen Focus". He spent almost three years doing research about why people can't focus deeply, and what to do to solve this problem. He went through the problem of the ADHD in kids, and he found out that overprotection and imprisonment are one of the main reasons that lead to this condition in kids. The solution that he suggested is to give children more "Free play time" without supervision because when a kid is freed from his parents' instructions, he is more open to learning, he will try to figure out things by himself, he will then develop a sense of self-reliance and self-confidence.

As a parent, you can still give your kid more free play time without him getting sick. There are a few simple tips and suggestions that you can follow like giving him a lunch box with gluten-free food, or inviting his friends to your house so you have more control on the dietary side, etc...

Mindset Point :

Prioritize your child's health and well-being over potential conflicts with relatives.

Now here 'is your "Children Stay Safe List":

- **Consider sending your kid with his own lunchbox to ensure she has safe food options.**
- **Teach your kid to say "no thank you" to foods she shouldn't have.**

- **Set boundaries to protect your kid if others don't understand or support his dietary needs.**

- **Provide a printout of foods you can or cannot have to help others understand your kid's dietary needs, or when he is leaving out with someone else than you.**

- **Prioritize safety and health above others' opinions or convenience.**

- Consider using visual aids like photos to show the effects of gluten consumption on your kid to increase awareness of your environment.

- Find gluten-free options at fast food places or specific locations to inform family members of where to bring your kid.

- Freeze extra gluten-free bread, cupcakes...and store them in the refrigerator to keep it fresh.

- Look for gluten-free recipes or pre-made options for your kid's favorite foods.

- Always carry safe snacks with you when going out.

- Ensure medications are gluten-free and communicate with pharmacists and distributors if needed.

- Start with simple, plain foods your kid enjoys, and get creative later.
- Consider using a grab bag with essential items to ensure your kid's safety and comfort when out.

- Gradually expose your kid to different environments and teach him how to keep himself safe.

- Empower your kid to be in control of her body and situation. You can buy him books on grit, self-confidence, etc...

- Be aware of the potential development of anxiety disorders with chronic medical conditions and address them early. Especially ADHD

Situation 2:

Who prepares the food?

I am the only gluten-sensitive person in a five-member family. I can manage my dietary preferences without constraining the whole family to live on gluten-free food. Most of the time I cook the food, and I rarely get contaminated. I follow simple hygiene smeasures that keep me safe from any symptom's triggers and cross-contamination factors. I will share them with you in a second along with other tricks. So, if you are asking if it is OK to cook gluten-containing food for your family, then the answer is yes as long as you take proper precautions. I have been doing this for years without problems, and I actually enjoy it!

If you can convince your family to eat (only) gluten-free food, then things will be much easier for you. As for me, I have chosen to make a little extra effort in food preparation to let them eat normally.

I want the kids to fully enjoy all sorts of food available to them, and I will share with you what I have learned to make this possible in case you want to take the same route. However, these tips are also extremely useful even if your whole family consumes only gluten-free. They will add an extra layer of protection and confidence to your daily life.

You can also refer to these tips if you are preparing food for a gluten-free person, like Laura who is not gluten-free, unlike her husband. She is a stay-at-home mom, and every morning she has to prepare sandwiches for her husband for his lunchtime at his workplace. Her husband was recently diagnosed with celiac, and she was looking for advice online when someone pointed her to our association. I wasn't there that day, but the advisor who spoke to her told me that her main struggle was how to manage the food preparation side. He then handed her the checklist I personally designed and made available for these situations. One month later, she visited us again along with her husband to thank us for that checklist, and to ask for guidance in other areas of their life.

Mindset Point :

Adopt a positive attitude towards cooking and enjoy the process. Start with small recipes, and get creative later

So here is your "Stay Safe List" while preparing gluten-free food:

- **Before preparing food, use warm water and gluten-free soap to clean the cooking area, including countertops, cutting boards, utensils, and any other surfaces that are in direct contact with food.**
- **Use separate utensils, cutting boards, pots, and pans dedicated to cook only gluten-free food.**
- **Avoid wooden utensils or porous materials that retain gluten particles. Use preferably stainless-steel material.**
- **Use labels to markup clearly gluten-free ingredients in the pantry and refrigerator, so you don't use the wrong ingredients accidently.**
- **Practice ingredient segregation to keep gluten-free and gluten-containing ingredients separate.**
- **Avoid using shared condiments like butter, spreads, sauces...and use separate containers or dispensers for them.**
- **Wash your hands thoroughly before and after handling gluten-containing ingredients.**
- **Wear gloves when handling gluten-containing food.**
- **Clean and sanitize surfaces, utensils, and cutting boards after each use.**

- If you can separate and dedicate a specific area in your kitchen to cook only gluten-free food, then do it.
- Use labeled bags, and containers to separate gluten free-food from other ingredients in the fridge.
- Use toaster bags if you don't have a separate toaster.
- Follow the tips in the "At the Grocery Chapter" to buy right food, and to protect yourself from cross-contamination before getting your food at the kitchen.

Situation 3:

How to enjoy your travel

My first trip after I was diagnosed with gluten intolerance was extremely challenging. Our company had a major project in a small town near Tennessee. I had to make 4 hour's travel by plane to attend the kick-off meeting with the partners we will work with, and then, I had to stay there for 2 days to make sure everything is going smoothly. I can say the flight time was OK because I had a big meal before getting on the plane. Once arrived, I bought some snacks and pre-made meals at the airport so I can eat them in the hotel, and then I headed up to the town.

The town was a small one, there were only two major groceries, and none of them was offering gluten-free food except some protein bars, and some snacks. I asked the hotel if they could offer a gluten-free menu, and I was faced with big opened eyes from the receptionist wondering what is gluten?! I just told him it was a kind of food allergy - I was really tired and stressed, so I didn't have the mood to give him an extensive explanation about gluten intolerance - He then called the Hotel chef, and asked him if he can accommodate my request, to my surprise, the chef knows what is gluten intolerance, he even mentioned gluten contamination, but the problem was he can only offer vegetables and some salads in the menu, and nothing more. He told me if I informed the hotel prior to my arrival about my dietary needs, he could accommodate me. That was my mistake, I admit it!

So for the next 2 days, I was feeding on veggies and some snacks. I was literally starving, lacking energy. I really had a difficult time keeping up with the business meetings, and the workload because I couldn't eat well.

That was the last time I have accepted to go on an unexpected business trip. I told my manager that if the company wanted to send me on a trip like this, they must inform me 48 h before, so I could have enough time to make my own preparations. I have asked my doctor to write me a letter explaining my health condition, which I handed to the administration as proof.

I learned the hard way that preparation and planning are the keys to a successful trip if you are gluten-free. I could prepare some food at home and take it with me. I could also check available restaurants that offer gluten-free menus in that town before landing in it. I could call the hotel and ask them to prepare gluten-free meals for my staying period...these are among many things I could do to make my travel time better.

I have learned through the course of the years some great tips through my personal experience, and through the experience of other people like us. Let me share them with you...

Mindset Point:

Your ability to adapt and manage the situation during your trip shows incredible resilience. Celebrate your strength and determination, as these qualities will continue to serve you well in various aspects of life.

Here is your "**Travel Stay Safe List**":

- **Planning ahead is crucial for individuals with gluten intolerance to avoid accidental gluten consumption.**

- **Use the "Find Me Gluten Free" app to find restaurants and places that offer gluten-free meals wherever you are.**

- **When traveling, pack your own food and utensils.**

- You may want to stay in Airbnbs or accommodations with kitchenettes to have control over their food preparation. You can use the available microwaves to heat your pre-made meals

- Bring small a cooler with ice packs, or utilize the hotel room's fridge to store your food safely for a long time.

- Contact the restaurant and speak to the cook who can provide assurance and information about gluten-free options.

- Eat a satisfying meal before traveling to help manage food concerns during the journey.

- Pack your own snacks for airport or flight travel. I found out that not all airports are gluten-free friendly.

- Check Google for restaurant websites and menus to get additional information about available gluten-free options. You can type in Google something like "Gluten-free restaurants near me"

- Carrying coffee mugs with heaters and warming carriers can be useful for heating gluten-free food while on the go.

- When traveling by plane, it is possible to bring certain foods like hard-boiled eggs, grilled chicken, quinoa, and cut-up veggies.

- Check with TSA (Transportation Security Administration), or call airport security directly about permitted food items you can carry into the airport without problems.

- Use insulated lunchboxes, and add ice to food after passing security checks.

- You can request a gluten-free meal ahead of time for in-flight meals.

- If you travel with a group of people, tell inform them about your dietary needs to find solutions that suit you and them.

- Before traveling to a destination, ask people in Facebook groups about places that offer gluten-free food in your destination. You will get insightful answers.

Situation 4:
Kiss without fear

I bet you will find the following fact hilarious, but it's true! Kissing may trigger your symptoms! Yep, you read it correctly. Did your partner just devoured something that had gluten in it without brushing his teeth? Then there is a -Tinny- chance of gluten contamination if you kiss him.

But hey, fear not! I've got some tips for you:

- Freshness wins, and gluten loses: Make sure your partner brushes his teeth or uses mouthwash before smooching.
- Gluten-Free Lip Service: Get your partner to use a gluten-free lip balm or lipstick.
- Discuss: Open up about your gluten intolerance with your smooch buddy. Communication is the gluten-free secret sauce!
- Gluten-digesting enzymes: These handy helpers can come to the rescue for small gluten mishaps. Talk to your healthcare provider about recommendations.

There are other behaviors like kissing that may trigger your symptoms, including:

Drinking after your husband/wife, child, or someone who is not gluten-free

Let someone drink from your bottle or cup

Communal snack bowls, buffet spreads, or potlucks during parties

Double-Dipping…

Mindset Point:

Openly discussing your gluten intolerance with your partner is a great step towards building a strong and supportive relationship. When you communicate your needs, you create an environment where both of you can work together to find solutions.

Now here is your "**Kissing Stay Safe list**":

- **Make sure your partner brushes his teeth before any intimate session.**

- **Use only gluten-free lipstick.**

- Create a gluten-free drink zone: When sharing drinks, use separate cups. You can also label your gluten-free beverages to avoid mix-ups.

- Bring Your Own Bottle: Carry your own water bottle, so you won't have to rely on using communal cups.

- Keep your snacks separate from others. You may pack individual portions, or use sealable containers to prevent contamination.

- Dipping Distinction: Opt for single-serve portions or use separate utensils for gluten-free options.

- Clear Communication: Clearly communicate your gluten intolerance to friends, family, and coworkers, so they understand your needs and support you.

- Potluck Precautions: Bring your own gluten-free dish that you can enjoy without worries.

- Just Ask: If you're unsure about the safety of a food or situation, it's okay to decline or ask questions. Remember, you are responsible for your own choices!

Situation 5:

Enjoy party time:

Three months after being diagnosed with gluten intolerance, I was invited to a birthday party. Everyone was having a great time, biting cakes and cookies, and exchanging conversations, except me! I was feeling left out, longing for a simple cookie to munch on. A young lady named Lise and her son approached me. Curious about my solitude, she gently asked why I wasn't joining in on the party fun.

I explained my gluten sensitivity and the dietary restrictions that came with it. To my surprise, Lise revealed that she, too, had celiac disease. But she had found a clever workaround! She either bakes gluten-free cupcakes at home or buys them from the grocery store and freezes them. Then, before events like this birthday party, she frosts them and brings them along. She actually reached into a bag she had brought and handed me one of them.

We spent most of the rest of the party together. She introduced me to her friends and handed me at the end of the party an invitation to join a gluten association that she was a member of. I have attended several meetings, learned a lot, and most importantly could connect with other people like me - I will come back to this point in detail in the upcoming chapters - Unfortunately, we moved to Chicago six months later!

I was grateful and excited at the same time, first because the cupcake was really tasty, and second because this little trick will let me enjoy future parties and birthdays like this with zero worry about gluten. It was a situation that clearly demonstrated that small tips and acts may help me to not let the gluten sensitivity control my life, or steal my moments of joy.

Mindset Point:

Focus on Solutions, Not Limitations: Instead of dwelling on the limitations imposed by gluten intolerance, concentrate on the solutions and possibilities available to you. Lise's simple act of sharing a cupcake opened up a world of opportunities for you to participate in future parties worry-free.

Here is your "**Stay Safe List**" to enjoy your time, and not feel isolated during parties:

- Bake cupcakes, tarts, or similar food and freeze them 2 or 3 days before going to a party. Take them out of the fridge 1 or 2 hours before leaving, and frost them if needed.

- If you are not in the mood to bake, or if you have several parties in a row and don't have enough time (or energy) to bake, then, buy them from your grocery store. Sometimes the grocery stores don't keep them on the front shelves because they don't sell so often. Just ask the grocery area supervisor, and he will point you out to where to find them.

- I suggest you put your cupcakes or tarts in ziploc bags prior to putting them in the fridge, it will protect them from humidity, cross-contamination, and from getting freezer burnt.

- If you have a loaf cake, or if you bought a large-size cake in a clamshell, then slice the cake into small portions, insert them into individual food bags, and freeze them. I found out this is the most practical way if you are not the only person in the house that needs gluten-free treats, or if you are planning a long trip, or if you have several parties in a small span of time. It is also a creative way to keep a large amount of cupcakes especially if you are planning to share them with other gluten-sensitive people (similar to what Lise did with me!)

- You can also get your local gluten-free bakery to deliver your cakes to you.

- Find additional tips related to parties in the "Stay Safe List" that you can find at the end of the "Kiss without fear" chapter.

Situation 6:

Precautions during a hospital stay

I had this major knee reconstruction surgery a while back. I was more concerned about the gluten-free food situation at the hospital than about the surgery itself! And I was right. It turned into a real gluten-filled nightmare during my stay there. I had heard those horror stories, and unfortunately, I had become one of them.

From day one, it was clear that the hospital staff didn't grasp the uniqueness of my dietary needs. When I asked about their gluten-free menu, I was met with blank stares and confusion. It was like I was speaking a foreign language. I was literally surprised to face this situation in a hospital!

From there, things were getting worse. The so-called "gluten-free" meals they provided were disastrous. I can't even call them proper food for humans. All I was served was some plain insufficiently steamed veggies, and a dry piece of chicken during my stay. This is not the kind of meal that's gonna help you to recover from surgery!

I talked to their so-called dietician, but it felt like my words were falling on deaf ears. They just didn't care, or at least that was my feeling back then. I encountered gluten in sauces, dressings, and even some of the medications they were administering. It was a real gluten minefield!

I ended up relying on the snacks I had packed as my saving grace. But still, it was disheartening to go through this in the very place that was supposed to be taking care of me.

Now, let me tell you what I learned from this. First off, be your own advocate. You've gotta speak up and make sure the hospital staff understands your dietary needs, even if it feels like you're repeating yourself a hundred times. Secondly, when you are gluten sensitive, then don't rely on the hospital's promises, period! Be prepared. Bring your own snacks and meals, or make someone bring them to you. It's better to be safe than sorry. Third, you are more likely to be the most knowledgeable person in the room about gluten intolerance. The nurses that take care of you, and the people in the kitchen in most cases don't have a clue about gluten sensitivity, or cross-contamination, so you have to clearly communicate your needs, and take your precautions.

And finally, I learned that not all hospitals are created equal. Do your research and find a hospital that truly understands and prioritizes your needs. Don't just assume they'll have it all figured out.

Note: As I wrote these lines, a friend of mine who has celiac was admitted to this same hospital for surgery, and she had to stay there for 2 days. I spoke to her over the phone about her experience in that hospital, especially their gluten-free menu! Seems like they now have a dedicated kitchen and dedicated cooking materials for people with specific needs like gluten intolerance. Good for them, and for people like us!

Before closing this chapter, I would like to ask you for a favor. If you could write a letter to your hospital after leaving, please do so. By doing so, you will actively contribute to the movement of raising awareness around our dietary needs. Your letter may be the reason other gluten intolerant and celiac disease people have better experiences when forced to spend time in hospitals.

If you have had a positive experience, write a letter to express your gratitude, encourage continual improvement, and thank the hospital staff that supported you with their attention, care, and compassion.

By contrast, if your days were not as you wanted, make your letter an advocate to share your experience, your feelings, maybe your anger, and suggestions for improvement. Hospital management appreciates this kind of feedback as it helps them improve their service, upgrade their overall quality, and stay close to their market's needs.

Mindset Point:

Being your own advocate is crucial, especially in situations where others may not fully understand your condition. Your determination to communicate your needs despite facing challenges is commendable.

Here's your **hospital "Stay Safe List"**:

- **Contact local celiac disease support organizations for recommendations on hospitals with good track records in accommodating gluten-free diets. You can also do research on the Internet, but I find out that asking on Facebook groups is the most effective and reliable way, as you can get quick and real feedback from real people.**

- Ask for a gluten-free menu, or talk to the hospital staff especially your doctor, the dietician, and the floor director on the unit you'll be recovering in.

- Ask the nursing staff to double-check your medications for potential gluten-containing ingredients.

- When you are served the food ask the person who brought it (or the people in the kitchen) how the food was prepared. Was it separated from the other food, or was it cooked it all together? A friend of mine asked this same question when she was served her gluten-free food, and the answer was: "It was prepared all together"! This is a cross-contamination you definitely want to avoid.

- Have a written list of safe and unsafe ingredients, food additives, and hidden sources of gluten to help you navigate food choices during your stay.

- Involve a trusted family member or friend who can advocate on your behalf regarding your dietary needs, especially if you're unable to communicate during your stay.

- Prepare a list of local gluten-free restaurants or delivery services that can provide safe meals if needed.

- Pack your own gluten-free snacks and meals to ensure you have safe options readily available.

- If possible, arrange for a family member or friend to bring you home-cooked gluten-free meals during your hospital stay.

- Stay hydrated and ensure any beverages served to you are free from gluten-containing additives or flavorings.

- Ask the hospital for a room with a fridge so you can keep your food in it, or bring a small fridge with you.

- Keep a food diary during your hospital stay, noting any symptoms or reactions you experience, to help identify any potential sources of gluten contamination.

- Consider wearing a medical alert bracelet or necklace indicating your celiac disease and gluten intolerance to alert healthcare providers.

- Take your gluten-free lotions and soap with you.

And here is a suggested list of foods to take with you if you are still not sure about the hospital you are going to stay in (See "Ready to go gluten-free foods and snacks" chapter for more suggestions)

- Gluten-free bread or wraps: Certified gluten-free, or homemade.
- Nut butter or seed butter: Peanut butter, almond butter, or sunflower seed butter to eat with gluten-free bread
- Nuts and seeds.
- Hard cooked eggs, applesauce & fruit
- Fresh fruits and vegetables: Pack a variety of fresh fruits and vegetables that are easy to consume and do not require refrigeration, such as apples, bananas, carrots, or snap peas.
- Gluten-free snacks: Like gluten-free granola bars, rice cakes, popcorn, or trail mix.
- Pre-packaged gluten-free meals: Microwavable rice bowls, gluten-free pasta dishes.
- Gluten-free protein sources: Pack canned tuna, salmon, chicken, as well as gluten-free jerky, protein bars.
- Gluten-free crackers or rice cakes: These can be enjoyed on their own or paired with spreads like hummus or dairy-free cheese.

- Gluten-free instant oatmeal or cereal: You can get hot water or milk from the hospital
- Gluten-free canned soups, chili, or quinoa, which can be prepared with hot water or in a microwave.
- Beverages: bottled water, herbal tea bags, or gluten-free instant coffee.

Situation 7:

How to stay safe at work :

One day we had a big meeting at the company I was working for. I was a project engineer back then, and I was an attendee.

I remember the heads of engineering, operations, and safety sections were all attending that meeting too, which meant some big decisions would be taken there. Fast forward, during the meeting we were served lunch boxes. There was meat, fruit, bread, and veggie salad. Of course, I couldn't eat anything of that including the salad because of possible cross-contamination.

Before that meeting took place, I have seen a post on Facebook of a lady that got fired because she was constantly sick for 6 months, and the reason is the food she got served by her company in a meeting, which was gluten contaminated.

I wanted to avoid being in a similar situation, so I pulled out a lettuce sandwich from my bag and started eating when the operations director asked if I didn't like the food the company served. I replied that I have a food allergy and I must be very careful about what I put in my mouth.

He then replied "Sorry to hear that, I didn't know it", then he took his pen, and noted something down in his notebook.

One week later, all the employees in the company received a form to fill in with information about their food allergies, and what type of food they could tolerate.

Later on, I learned from my direct manager that the operations director wrote was about how to accommodate food allergies when serving food to people at meetings! I was surprised to learn that because I didn't expect it by any means. I have heard completely different stories from some friends. Some people fought with their managers because they forced them to eat the food served in a meeting, and others were harassed because of that!

My company was a big player in the field of construction, they had the human, financial, and logistical means to accommodate people's dietary needs during assemblies. I understand that this is not applicable to everyone, and more likely you have to take care of yourself during your working hours, and I have some tips that could help you!

I want to add that I had to make some trips from the office to the construction sites back and forth several times during the month, so I feel your struggle if your job requires you to be constantly on the road, or to make frequent visits to customers, and I have also some tips for you too!

Sticking to these tips and to the other tips in this book has helped me to stay in good health and mood over the course of the years. I got sick sometimes, and I didn't know why. Maybe I ate some food with hidden gluten, maybe someone touched my food while I was absent, or maybe I ignored basic safety measures, who knows? Probably that will also happen to you, but it will be very rare, and when this occurs, just take a day or two off, or talk to your manager about working from home, or negotiate flexible working hours... and believe me, this is the best you can do when you get contaminated, rather than making mistakes because of lack of focus and pain.

Mindset Point:

Keep an eye out for potential improvements in the workplace that can benefit both yourself and others. Being proactive in suggesting positive changes can make a significant impact on company culture.

So here is your "**Stay safe list at work**":

- **Pack gluten-free lunch with options like salads, fruits, protein bars, etc...if you need ideas about** foods/snacks you can pack, then please check the chapter " Foods & Snacks Ideas "

- Buy a small cooler with blue ice blocks to keep lunch and drinks cold while out. Keep the cooler in your car, or truck if you are a truck driver.

- Snack options for on-the-go: nuts/trail mix, jerky (soy sauce-free), popcorn, chips, Kind bars, veggie straws, meat and cheese roll-ups, and fruits.

- Eat well before going to a meeting.

- Pack meals for work using a lunchbox with a mini–ice pack for salads, berries, or cold items.

- Communicate your dietary needs to your employer to ensure gluten-free meals are provided at work.

- Keep in your bag an anti-gluten enzyme for a quick fix in case you get contaminated accidentally at work.

- Bring your own water bottle with you. You may put a sticker on the bottle to prevent other people from using it in your absence, or just keep it in your drawer when you are not around your desk.

- **Always wash your hands very well before eating lunch at work, or when you are outside, and don't use the hand sanitizers provided by your company as they contain gluten. Bring your own hand sanitizer.**

- **If you have to keep your lunch in the common fridge provided by the company, then, always use food plastic bags to cover it, and protect it from cross-contamination.**

- **To avoid getting contaminated by other people's food, always eat on a towel that protects your food from being on direct contact with the surface.**

Here are some food & snacks ideas for you to enjoy during working hours (**you can find more ideas in the chapter "Food and Snacks ideas"**):

- Almond Flour Chocolate Chip Cookies
- Chocolate Covered Rice Cakes
- Pasta Salad
- Turkey or Ham Roll-Ups with Cheese
- Salad with Turkey and Cheese
- Sliced Apples or Banana with Nut Butter
- Olives
- Cheese
- GF (gluten-free) lunch meats (smoked turkey, ham)

- GF beet crackers
- Almonds
- Cashews
- Asiago artichoke dip
- Carrots
- Celery
- Yogurt with GF granola
- Pineapple
- Watermelon
- Grapes
- Dried apricots
- GF protein bars
- GF oats
- Frozen pomegranate
- Cinnamon
- Veggies
- Hummus
- Deli meat
- Fresh fruit
- Nuts/trail mix
- Jerky (ensure no soy sauce)
- Skinny Pop/popcorn
- Quest tortilla chips
- Kind bars
- Veggie straws
- Meat & cheese rollups

- Bite-sized fruit
- Quest brand bars
- Almond flour chocolate chip cookies
- Chocolate-covered rice cakes
- Cucumbers
- GF lunch salad with turkey and cheese
- GF pasta
- Olives
- Tomatoes
- Celery
- Sliced apples
- Banana
- Nut butter
- Chomps jerky
- Apple
- Orange
- Canned sardines or tuna
- Salad
- Berries
- Drink mixes
- Protein powders
- Dried fruit
- Rice cakes
- GF fruit jerky
- GF crackers with nut butter
- GF nuts

Situation 8:

How to do your grocery :

Doing grocery as a newly diagnosed gluten-sensitive person used to be a painful time for me. I remember spending over 3 hours at the local store looking for gluten-free food, reading labels, and verifying every single ingredient on Google. By the time I wrote these lines, things had gotten much better, easier, and affordable.

I have three rules I never infringe upon when I want to do my GF grocery. These rules allow me to spend much less time and money on my gluten-free grocery, and make the whole experience enjoyable and stress-free. The rules are:

1. Planning

2. Eat less processed food

3. Don't waste

Planning is truly the key to making your grocery trip successful, especially if you have to travel for more than 1 hour to reach the nearest store that offers gluten-free food. I start planning by making a meal plan for the whole week. During busy weeks, I plan to cook for three days only, and I use what is left over for the remaining days. For example, I cook extra food on Monday, put it in the fridge what is left over to eat on Tuesday, cook again on Wednesday, and eat what's left over on Thursday. I start meal planning by checking the fridge, freezer, and pantry to see if anything is missing. I also check to see if there is something I don't have to buy for the upcoming week. I usually do this on Sunday. I set aside 20 minutes in the morning to make a grocery list to have enough time to cook dinner with the ingredients I bought that day.

At the grocery store, I stick to my list to avoid getting distracted and minimize my time there. I rarely purchase processed food unless it is required for a recipe, or if I have to prepare something special like cakes or tarts. I also use a barcode scanner app that helps me spot any gluten-contaminated products, which saves me from the hassle of reading food ingredients, and I do it for all processed food including the labeled "gluten-free" ones. I focus on naturally gluten-free foods like fruits, eggs, meats, vegetables, rice, and potatoes...these foods tend to be less expensive and healthier than processed ones.

Finally, I purchase some toaster bags to avoid getting gluten contaminated in case I have to travel or use the toast maker at the office.

<u>Mindset Point:</u>

As you continue to explore gluten-free options, stay open to trying new products or brands. You might discover some hidden gems that become staples in your grocery list.

Here is your " **Stay Safe List for Grocery Time**":

- **Always make a weekly meal plan before grocery shopping. Take 20 minutes in the morning to do it.**

- **Check your freezer, fridge, and pantry before making your grocery list for the week.**

- **Make a weekly grocery list, take it with you, and stick to it!**

- **Use a barcode scanner app to help you spot and avoid gluten-containing foods.**

- **Focus on naturally gluten-free foods like meats, vegetables, rice, and potatoes. Purchase at the perimeter of the store where you can find fresh food.**

- **Cook extra food and freeze it for later use. No waste!**

- **Decrease your gluten-free bill by limiting your intake of processed and canned food.**

- **Invest in GF cookbooks or find recipes online to cook your own food. Start with easy egg recipes, and get creative slowly.**

- **Look at online recipes to make your own seasonings and dressings to avoid hidden resources of gluten. You will get less sick, and you will have more money to invest in other things.**

- **Save leftover vegetables and meats in the freezer for quick soups.**

- **Request a gluten-free food list from customer service at stores.**

Situation 9:

How to stay safe when using Cosmetics:

Cosmetic and beauty products may represent symptoms triggers if you are gluten sensitive or if you have celiac. Even though there is no global agreement about the possibility of gluten absorption through the skin, there is a considerable fraction of people who get sick as soon as they touch something that contains gluten, I have met them, I saw their stories online, and I can tell you with confidence that their struggles are real.

If you stick to a gluten-free diet, and if you are confident in your precautions but you still get some symptoms like itchy skin, migraines, and other gluten attacks, then you should question your beauty and cosmetic products, especially if you are a woman, or if you are involved in an environment or situation that requires direct contact with these products like weddings, TV plateaux, the healthcare environment, Spa, and so on...

If you have doubts about whether cosmetic products are the source of your bad moments or not, then, what you have to do is pay close attention to your body's reaction after using them. Any type of reaction means you belong to the group of people who may get sick through their skin. In this case, switch to gluten-free cosmetics. I would suggest not applying lipstick or balm, or any cosmetic product to lips during this test, because these products may get accidentally absorbed through your mouth, causing some reactions, and you will wrongly think that the responsible is other skin care or cosmetic products.

There are several cosmetic brands that produce gluten-free products. I know many women that are using them on a daily basis, and they are happy with them. I advise you to do your own research and find the ones that suit you. You will find some tips at the end of this chapter that will help you navigate these products safely to choose the right ones. I had planned to list some brands in this book as a reference not only for the cosmetics side, but for all categories including food, beverages, snacks, etc…, however, the process of validating and verifying each one of them has taken more time than I have expected, so I decided to include them in the next edition of this book.

Mindset Point:

If you are sensitive to gluten-containing cosmetics, it's fine, you are not the only one. Instead, look at this

situation as an opportunity to discover new brands and options that will make you feel even better.

Here is your "**Stay Safe List for Cosmetics**":

- **Watch your body's reactions closely after applying cosmetics. If you have gluten attacks, switch to gluten-free brands.**

- **Avoid applying cosmetics in areas close to your mouth and nose.**

- **Your cosmetics brand will more likely have an 800 number that you can call if you have any doubt or questions about a specific product. Use it!**

- **Avoid using products from non-recognizable brands**

- **Look for brands recommendations online, especially in gluten-specific groups.**

- **Before fully applying a new cosmetic product to your skin, perform a patch test on a small area of the skin to check for any adverse reactions or sensitivities.**

- **Use a label-scanning app to detect and avoid cosmetics with gluten**

- **Use mineral-based cosmetics as they tend to be less contaminated.**

- **Avoid cosmetics with hidden gluten sources. Here is a list of some of the hidden resources that may be found in cosmetics:**

  - Avena Sativa (Oat) Bran
  - Avena Sativa (Oat) Kernel Extract
  - Avena Sativa (Oat) Kernel Flour
  - Barley Flour
  - Barley Grass
  - Dextrin (unless specified as gluten-free)
  - Hordeum Vulgare (Barley) Extract
  - Hordeum Vulgare (Barley) Flour
  - Hordeum Vulgare (Barley) Grass Powder
  - Hydrolyzed Barley Protein
  - Hydrolyzed Oat Protein
  - Hydrolyzed Rye Protein
  - Hydrolyzed Wheat Protein
  - Malt Extract
  - Maltodextrin (unless specified as gluten-free)
  - Oat Beta-Glucan
  - Rye Flour
  - Secale Cereale (Rye) Seed Extract
  - Secale Cereale (Rye) Seed Flour

- Triticum Vulgare (Wheat) Bran
- Triticum Vulgare (Wheat) Bran Extract
- Triticum Vulgare (Wheat) Germ Extract
- Triticum Vulgare (Wheat) Germ Oil
- Triticum Vulgare (Wheat) Germ Powder
- Wheat Bran Extract
- Wheat Germ Oil
- Wheat Starch

Situation 10:
Takeout and delivery

Sometimes I use takeout and delivery services to get my gluten-free food delivered. Here are some guidelines for using them properly as a gluten-sensitive person:

- **Choose only gluten-free restaurants**: Make sure to select restaurants that specifically offer gluten-free options on their menu. You can find these restaurants by asking other people directly or via Facebook groups.
- **Check the Menu and Ingredients**: Thoroughly review the menu and ingredient list provided by the restaurant to make sure they suit your sensitivity, especially if you have other allergies.
- **Communicate Your Dietary Needs**: When placing your order, clearly communicate that you have gluten sensitivity. Request that your meal be prepared separately from gluten-containing dishes to avoid cross-contamination.
- **Check the restaurant's website**: Don't hesitate to check the website of the restaurant to verify the precautions taken to prevent cross-contamination and the food preparation process.
- **Read Reviews and Ratings**: Before ordering from a new restaurant, check online reviews and ratings to see

if other gluten-sensitive customers have had positive experiences with their gluten-free options.
- **Double-Check Delivery Instructions**.
- **Inspect the Order Upon Delivery**: When your food arrives, check the order to ensure that it's correct and that all the items are indeed gluten-free. If something looks suspicious, contact the restaurant immediately.
- **Keep Emergency Gluten-Free Snacks**: While most restaurants do their best to provide safe gluten-free options, it's a good idea to have some emergency gluten-free snacks at home, just in case the delivered order isn't as expected.
- **Feedback and Loyalty Programs**: If you have a positive experience, consider providing feedback to the restaurant. Some places offer loyalty programs for frequent customers, which might be beneficial for your future gluten-free orders.
- **Plan Ahead**: Delivery times can vary, so plan your order in advance, especially if you have specific meal times or events you need to cater to.
- **Use Reputable Delivery Apps or Websites**: Opt for well-known and reputable delivery apps or websites that allow you to filter restaurants based on their gluten-free options. This can help you find suitable places more easily.
- **Look for Certified Gluten-Free Labels**: Some restaurants or food items may have gluten-free certifications from recognized organizations. These

certifications can give you more confidence in the safety of your order.

- **Avoid Common Gluten-Containing Items**: Be cautious of common gluten-containing ingredients like wheat, barley, rye, and their derivatives. Double-check if any sauces, dressings, or marinades are gluten-free.
- **Notify About Allergies**: Apart from your gluten sensitivity, if you have any other food allergies, ensure you communicate them clearly when placing your order.
- **Ask for Separate Packaging**: Request that your gluten-free items be packed separately from any gluten-containing items in your order. This helps reduce the risk of accidental contamination during transit.
- **Check for Customization Options**: Some restaurants may allow you to customize your order. Use this feature to remove any gluten-containing ingredients or ask for gluten-free alternatives.
- **Be Aware of Gluten Cross-Contamination**: Cross-contamination can occur during food preparation, cooking, and packaging. Seek restaurants that take cross-contamination seriously and follow strict protocols.
- **Keep an Eye on Portion Sizes**: Gluten-free dishes may sometimes come in smaller portions compared to regular dishes. Verify the portion sizes to ensure you're ordering enough to satisfy your hunger.

- **Save Allergy Cards or Notes**: If you have a written card or note detailing your gluten sensitivity and dietary requirements, save a digital copy on your phone. This way, you can easily share it with the restaurant if needed.
- **Track Your Orders**: Keep a record of the restaurants you've tried, their gluten-free offerings, and your experiences. This helps you remember which places you can trust for future orders.
- **Be Patient and Understanding**: While most restaurants strive to provide the best service, mistakes can happen. Be patient and understanding if there are occasional errors, but don't hesitate to reach out to address any concerns.
- **Keep a note of the restaurants** that you have had a positive experience with for future orders.
- **Share**: share the names of restaurants that you had a positive experience with.
- **Use Truspilot**: before ordering from a restaurant, search it on truspilot.com to see what other users are saying, especially if you will place a big order.

Situation 11:

Sport and outdoors activities

The following guidelines are recommended if you are planning an outdoor activity like camping, or going to the beach.

- **Plan Ahead**: Planning is the key, prior to going out, look nearby the location of activities for gluten-free dining options to ensure you have safe food choices.
- **Pack Gluten-Free Snacks**: Always carry gluten-free snacks with you, such as nuts, fruits, gluten-free energy bars, or rice cakes.
- **Stay Hydrated**: Bring a refillable water bottle to stay hydrated during activities. Dehydration can worsen the effects of gluten sensitivity, so drinking plenty of water is essential. Put a sticker on your bottle to prevent others from using it which may cause cross-contamination.
- **Inform Activity Leaders**: If you're participating in organized sports or guided outdoor activities, inform the leaders about your gluten sensitivity. They can assist in making appropriate arrangements or suggestions.

- **Bring your own material**: If you're cooking or grilling food during camping or picnics, then, use separate utensils and surfaces to avoid gluten exposure.
- **Communicate with Others**: If you're in a group setting, let your companions know about your gluten sensitivity and its importance. They can help you find suitable food options and be mindful of your needs.
- **First Aid Kit**: Carry a small first aid kit with essentials like gluten-free pain relievers, gluten-free enzymes, and any personal medications you may need.
- **Choose Safe Activities**: Engage in sports and activities that suit your fitness level and health condition. Avoid overexertion, especially if you are new to these activities.
- **Ask for advice on gluten-sensitivity groups**: you will get valuable feedback from other gluten-sensitive people.
- **Gluten-Free Restaurants and Apps**: Use smartphone apps or websites that can help you find gluten-free restaurants and eateries in the area you'll be visiting.
- **Be Cautious with Sauces and Condiments**: Be wary of sauces, dressings, and condiments, as they may contain gluten. Ask for gluten-free options or bring your own.

- **Educate Your Companions**: Profit from your activities to educate others about gluten intolerance, you can wear T-shirts, hats,...to spread the word about it.
- **Gluten-Free Sunscreen and Personal Care Products**: Check the ingredients in sunscreen and personal care products to ensure they are gluten-free.
- **Inform Accommodation Providers**: If you're staying in a hotel or vacation rental, inform the staff about your gluten sensitivity in advance. Many accommodations are willing to accommodate special dietary needs.
- **Pack Wet Wipes and Hand Sanitizer**: Pack your own gluten-free soap and hand sanitizers.
- **Carry Gluten-Free Food Cards**: If you're traveling to a region with a different language, consider carrying food cards in the local language that explain your dietary restrictions. This can help you communicate your needs more effectively.
- **Gluten-Free Camping Meals**: If you're camping, prepare gluten-free meals in advance and pack them in sealed containers to avoid cross-contamination.
- **Mindful Picnics**: If having a picnic, use separate containers for gluten-free and gluten-containing foods, and be cautious when sharing utensils or plates.

Ready to go gluten-free foods & snacks

- All the fruit
- All the veggies
- Almond butter
- Almond flour chocolate chip cookies
- Almond flour crackers
- Almonds
- Apple
- Apple slices
- Applesauce
- Asiago artichoke dip
- Avocado
- Baby bell
- Baby bell cheese
- Baby carrots
- Bagels
- Bags of popcorn
- Banana
- Beef jerky
- Berries
- Bite-sized fruit
- Black coffee
- Blueberries
- Broccoli salad
- Canned beans
- Canned beans (cannelini, garbanzo, kidney)
- Canned sardines or tuna

- canned tuna,
- Carrots
- Carrots with ranch dressing
- Cashews
- Celery
- Celery sticks
- Cheese
- Cheese cubes
- Cheese roll ups
- Cheese sticks
- Cheese sticks (baby bell cheese)
- Chia pudding
- Chicken for tacos
- Chicken salad
- chicken,
- Chips
- Chips and dip
- Choc chips
- Chocolate covered mango
- Chocolate Covered Rice Cakes
- Chocolate-covered mango
- Chocolate-covered rice cakes
- Chocolates
- Chomps jerky
- Cinnamon
- Coconut flakes
- Cold oatmeal yogurt
- Cold oatmeal yogurt or chia pudding with berries
- Corn tortilla
- Crackers

- Cream cheese
- Cubed avocado
- Cucumber
- Cucumber and tomato salad
- Cucumbers
- Curds
- Curry leaves
- Cut up fruit
- Cut up veggies
- Dairy-free cheeses
- Dairy-free yogurt
- Dairy-free yogurts
- Deli meat
- Deli meats
- Dried apricots
- Dried fruit
- Dried ice
- Dried pepperoni
- Drink mixes
- Egg salad
- Flank or skirt steak
- Flavored almonds
- Fresh fruit
- Frozen pomegranate
- Fruit
- Fruit (various types)
- GF (gluten-free) lunch meats (smoked turkey, ham)
- GF bagels
- GF beet crackers
- GF crackers
- GF crackers with nut butter

- GF fruit jerky
- GF lunch salad with turkey and cheese
- GF muffins
- GF nuts
- GF oats
- GF pasta
- GF protein bars
- Gf sandwich
- GF Snyder's pretzels
- GF sweet treat
- GF syders pretzels
- Gluten-free bread
- Gluten-free bread
- Gluten-free canned soups, chili, or quinoa (can be prepared with hot water or in a microwave).
- Gluten-free crackers
- gluten-free instant coffee.
- Gluten-free instant oatmeal or cereal (can be prepared with hot water or milk).
- gluten-free jerky,
- Gluten-free wraps
- Granola bars
- Grapes
- Grapples
- Green Apples w/ nut butter
- Grill flank or skirt steak
- Gummi candy

- Gummi candy/sweet treat (gluten-free)
- Ham
- Ham and cheese roll-ups
- Hamburger in a lettuce wrap (gluten-free)
- Hard boiled eggs
- **Hard-cooked eggs,**
- Hardboiled eggs
- Healthy GF muffins
- **herbal tea bags,**
- Homemade onion dip
- Homemade ranch dip
- Honey
- Hot dogs
- Hot green tea
- Hummus
- Hummus with baby carrots and the mini cucumbers
- Jelly
- Jerky
- Jerky (ensure no soy sauce)
- Kind bars
- Lemon
- Lettuce leaves
- Lettuce wrap
- Licorice (gluten-free, if available)
- Licorice (gluten-free)
- Luna Bars
- Lunch meat
- Mac n cheese cups
- Mac n cheese cups (gluten-free)

- Mayo
- Meat & cheese rollups
- Melons
- Merkt's port wine cheese
- Mini cucumbers
- Nut butter
- Nuts
- Nuts mixes
- Nuts/trail mix
- Olives
- Onion dip
- Orange
- Oven roasted turkey
- Pasta Salad
- Peanut butter
- Peanuts
- Pickle
- Pickle rolls
- Pineapple
- Pistachios
- Popcorn
- Portable charcuterie box
- Potatoes chips
- Pre-packaged gluten-free meals (e.g., microwavable rice bowls, gluten-free pasta dishes).
- Pretzels
- Protein bars
- Protein bars (gluten-free)
- protein bars)
- Protein powders

- Protein shake
- Pumpkin seeds
- Quest brand bars
- Quest cookies
- Quest tortilla chips
- Quick meal
- Raisins
- Ranch dressing
- Rice cakes
- Rice crackers
- Rice crackers or rice cakes
- Rice flakes
- Rice flakes (gluten-free)
- Rosemary crackers
- Salad
- Salad with Turkey and Cheese
- Salami
- Salami sticks
- salmon,
- Salted almonds
- Sandwiches
- Sandwiches pre-made with gluten-free bread
- Seed butter
- Skinny Pop/popcorn
- Sliced apples
- Sliced Apples or Banana with Nut Butter
- Smoothies
- Sparkling water
- Spices
- String cheese
- Stuffed celery

- sunflower seed butter
- Sunflower seeds
- Tangerines
- Tomato salad
- Tomatoes
- Trail mix
- Trail mix (peanuts, raisins, M&Ms)
- Tuna
- Tuna pouches
- Tuna salad
- Turkey or Ham Roll-Ups with Cheese
- Various nuts
- Veggie straws
- Veggies (various types)
- Watermelon
- Wraps
- Yogurt
- Yogurt with GF granola

Gluten free food & grocery list :

The following pages should be used as guide to help you with your grocery, and meal planning. Here is how to use them:

1. The foods in this list are gluten-free

2. All fresh fruits and vegetables are naturally gluten-free, hence, I did not mention them in these lists.

3. The foods in each category are alphabetically arranged.

4. For canned foods, always read the labels or use a barcode scanner to ensure they don't contain gluten.

Albacore Tuna	Halibut	Sardine
Amberjack	Hard Clam	Sauger
Anchovy	Herring	Scallops
Arctic Char	Jacksmelt	Sea Bass
Atlantic Cod	King Crab	Sea Urchin
Atlantic Croaker	King Mackerel	Shad
Atlantic Herring	Kingfish	Shark
Atlantic Mackerel	Lake Herring	Shrimp
Atlantic Salmon	Lake Trout	Silver Hake
Atlantic Scallops	Lake Whitefish	Silver Salmon
Barramundi	Lemon Sole	Skate
Bass	Lingcod	Smelt
Black Cod	Little Neck Clam	Snapper
Black Sea Bass	Lobster	Snow Crab
Blue Crab	Longfin Squid	Sole
Blue Marlin	Longnose Sucker	Spanish Mackerel
Bluefin Tuna	Mackerel	Spearfish
Bluefish	Mahi Mahi	Spot
Bonito	Monkfish	Spot Prawn
Bowfin	Mullet	Spotted Sea Trout
Branzino	Mussel	Squid
Brook Trout	Northern Pike	Steelhead Trout
Burbot	Octopus	Striped Bass
California Halibut	Oyster	Sturgeon
Carp	Pacific Cod	Surf Clam
Catfish	Pacific Halibut	Swordfish
Channel Catfish	Pacific Herring	Threadfin Shad
Chilean Sea Bass	Pacific Mackerel	Tilapia
Chinook Salmon	Pacific Rockfish	Tilefish
Chub Mackerel	Perch	Triggerfish
Cisco	Pike	Trout
Clam	Pink Salmon	Tuna
Cod	Pink Shrimp	Turbot
Coho Salmon	Pinto Abalone	Wahoo
Conch	Pollock	Walleye
Corvina	Pompano	Weakfish
Crab	Porgy	White Sucker
Crawfish	Rainbow Trout	Whitefish
Croaker	Red Snapper	Whiting
Cusk	Redfish	Yellow Perch
Cuttlefish	Rock Crab	Yellowfin Grouper
Dungeness Crab	Rock Lobster	Yellowfin Tuna
Eel	Rock Shrimp	Yellowtail
European Anchovy	Rockfish	
European Seabass	Round Goby	
Flounder	Round Scad	
Freshwater Eel	Round Whitefish	
Grouper	Sablefish	
Gulf Shrimp	Salmon	
Haddock	Sand Crab	

Acorn flour	Lupin flour
Adzuki bean flour	Macadamia flour
Almond flour	Mesquite flour
Amaranth flour	Millet flour
Arrowroot flour/starch	Mung bean flour
Artichoke flour	Mushroom flour
Asparagus flour	Navy bean flour
Banana flour	Oat flour (if certified gluten-free)
Beet flour	Onion flour
Black bean flour	Parsley flour
Breadfruit flour	Pea flour
Broccoli flour	Pecan flour
Brown rice flour	Pistachio flour
Buckwheat flour	Polenta
Cabbage flour	Popcorn flour
Carrot flour	Potato flour
Cassava flour	Pumpkin flour
Cauliflower flour	Pumpkin seed flour
Chard flour	Quinoa flour
Chestnut flour	Radicchio flour
Chia flour	Radish flour
Chickpea flour	Red bean flour
Coconut flour	Rice flour
Collard flour	Scallion flour
Corn flour	Sesame seed flour
Cornmeal	Shallot flour
Dandelion flour	Sorghum flour
Endive flour	Soursop flour
Escarole flour	Soy flour (if certified gluten-free)
Fava bean flour	Spinach flour
Flaxseed flour	Squash flour
Garbanzo bean flour	Sunflower seed flour
Garlic flour	Sweet lupin flour
Ginger flour	Sweet potato flour
Green banana flour	Tapioca flour/starch
Hazelnut flour	Teff flour
Hemp flour	Teff flour
Jackfruit flour	Tigernut flour
Kale flour	Walnut flour
Leek flour	Watercress flour
Lentil flour	White rice flour
Lettuce flour	Wild rice flour
Lima bean flour	Yucca flour
Lotus seed flour	Zucchini flour

- Amaranth pasta
- Artichoke pasta
- Bean thread noodles
- Black bean and brown rice pasta
- Black bean pasta
- Brown rice and almond pasta
- Brown rice and amaranth pasta
- Brown rice and black bean pasta
- Brown rice and black sesame pasta
- Brown rice and chestnut pasta
- Brown rice and chickpea pasta
- Brown rice and coconut pasta
- Brown rice and green tea pasta
- Brown rice and hemp pasta
- Brown rice and kale pasta
- Brown rice and millet pasta
- Brown rice and pumpkin pasta
- Brown rice and quinoa pasta
- Brown rice and red pepper pasta
- Brown rice and saffron pasta
- Brown rice and spinach pasta
- Brown rice and sweet potato pasta
- Brown rice and turmeric pasta
- Brown rice and walnut pasta
- Brown rice pasta
- Buckwheat and beetroot pasta
- Buckwheat and nettle pasta
- Buckwheat and onion pasta
- Buckwheat and sweet potato pasta
- Buckwheat pasta
- Chickpea and brown rice pasta
- Chickpea and lentil pasta
- Chickpea and quinoa pasta
- Chickpea and spinach pasta
- Chickpea pasta
- Corn and basil pasta
- Corn and chestnut pasta
- Corn and fava bean pasta
- Corn and pumpkin pasta
- Corn and quinoa pasta
- Corn and sesame pasta
- Corn and tomato pasta
- Corn pasta
- Edamame pasta
- Green pea and quinoa pasta
- Green pea pasta
- Kelp noodles
- Konjac noodles
- Lentil and brown rice pasta
- Lentil pasta
- Millet pasta
- Potato pasta
- Quinoa and almond pasta
- Quinoa and chestnut pasta
- Quinoa and chia pasta
- Quinoa and coconut pasta
- Quinoa and corn pasta
- Quinoa and hemp pasta
- Quinoa and kale pasta
- Quinoa and red pepper pasta
- Quinoa and saffron pasta
- Quinoa and spinach pasta
- Quinoa and sweet potato pasta
- Quinoa and turmeric pasta
- Quinoa and walnut pasta
- Quinoa pasta
- Red lentil and quinoa pasta
- Red lentil and sweet potato pasta
- Red lentil pasta
- Shirataki noodles
- Soba noodles (if made with 100% buckwheat)
- Sorghum pasta
- Soy and sweet potato pasta (if certified gluten-free)
- Soy pasta (if certified gluten-free)
- Spaghetti squash pasta
- Sweet potato and almond pasta
- Sweet potato and buckwheat pasta
- Sweet potato and chestnut pasta
- Sweet potato and coconut pasta
- Sweet potato and hemp pasta
- Sweet potato and kale pasta
- Sweet potato and red pepper pasta
- Sweet potato and turmeric pasta
- Sweet potato pasta
- Tapioca pasta
- Wild rice pasta
- Zucchini pasta

- Ajwain seeds
- Allspice berries
- Almond flour
- Almonds
- Amaranth
- Amaranth seeds
- Anise powder (anise seeds)
- Anise seeds
- Arrowroot
- Basil seeds
- Black cumin seeds
- Black pepper seeds
- Black sesame seeds
- Brazil nuts
- Brown mustard seeds
- Buckwheat
- Buckwheat groats
- Cacao nibs
- Caraway powder (caraway seeds)
- Caraway seeds
- Cardamom pods
- Cashews
- Cassava flour
- Celery seeds
- Chestnut flour
- Chia seeds
- Chickpea flour
- Coconut
- Coconut flour
- Coriander leaves (cilantro seeds)
- Coriander powder (coriander seeds)
- Coriander seeds
- Corn
- Cumin powder (cumin seeds)
- Cumin seeds
- Dill seeds
- Fava bean flour
- Fennel leaves (fennel seeds)
- Fennel powder (fennel seeds)
- Fennel seeds
- Fenugreek powder (fenugreek seeds)
- Flaxseeds
- Green peppercorns
- Hazelnut flour
- Hazelnuts
- Hemp hearts
- Hemp seeds
- Hulled hemp seeds
- Juniper berries
- Kalonji seeds (nigella seeds)
- Lentil flour
- Macadamia nuts
- Millet
- Millet seeds
- Mustard leaves (mustard seeds)
- Mustard powder (mustard seeds)
- Mustard seeds
- Nigella seeds
- Nutmeg seeds.
- Oats (if certified gluten-free)
- Papaya seeds
- Pecans
- Pepitas (pumpkin seeds without the shell)
- Pine nuts
- Pink peppercorns
- Pistachios
- Pomegranate seeds
- Popcorn
- Poppy seeds
- Potato flour
- Pumpkin seeds
- Quinoa
- Quinoa seeds
- Rice
- Rosemary seeds
- Safflower seeds
- Sage seeds
- Sesame paste (tahini)
- Sesame seeds
- Sesame tahini (ground sesame seeds)
- Sichuan peppercorns
- Sorghum
- Sorghum seeds
- Soy flour
- Star anise
- Sunflower butter (ground sunflower seeds)
- Sunflower seed butter
- Sunflower seeds
- Sweet potato flour
- Tahini (ground sesame seeds)
- Tapioca
- Teff
- Teff seeds
- Thyme seeds
- Toasted sesame seeds
- Toasted sunflower seeds
- Vanilla beans
- Walnuts
- Watermelon seed butter
- Watermelon seeds
- White pepper seeds
- Wild rice

- Alligator meat
- Beef
- Beef brisket
- Beef liver
- Beef ribs
- Beef sirloin
- Beef tenderloin
- Beef tongue
- Bison meat
- Chicken
- Chicken breast
- Chicken drumsticks
- Chicken hearts.
- Chicken legs
- Chicken liver
- Chicken liver pate
- Chicken thighs
- Chicken wings
- Clams
- Cornish hen meat
- Crab
- Duck liver
- Elk
- Elk meat
- Emu meat
- Goat
- Goat chops
- Goat shoulder
- Goat stew meat
- Goose
- Goose breast
- Goose legs
- Goose liver
- Ground beef
- Ground chicken
- Ground lamb
- Ground pork
- Ground turkey
- Grouse
- Grouse meat
- Guinea fowl
- Guinea fowl meat
- Kangaroo
- Kangaroo meat
- Lamb
- Lamb chops
- Lamb leg
- Lamb ribs
- Lamb shank
- Lamb shoulder
- Lobster meat
- Moose meat
- Mussels
- Octopus
- Ostrich meat
- Oysters
- Partridge meat
- Pheasant
- Quail meat
- Rabbit meat
- Scallops
- Shrimp meat
- Squid
- Turkey
- Turkey breast
- Turkey legs
- Turtle
- Turtle meat
- Venison
- Venison stew meat
- Wild boar

- Acai berries
- Acorns
- Adzuki beans
- Almond butter
- Almonds
- Amaranth
- Beech nuts
- Bitter nuts
- Black beans
- Black walnuts
- Brazil nuts
- Broad beans
- Buckwheat
- Butter beans
- Butternuts
- Cannellini beans
- Cashew butter
- Cashews
- Cedar nuts
- Chestnuts
- Chia seeds
- Chickpeas
- Chinkapins
- Chinquapins
- Cocoa beans
- Coconut
- Coquito nuts
- Fava beans
- Filberts
- Flaxseeds
- Garbanzo beans
- Gingko nuts
- Hazelnut butter
- Hazelnuts
- Hemp seeds
- Hickory nuts
- Horse chestnuts
- Indian nuts
- Java almonds
- Karuka nuts
- Kidney beans
- Kola nuts
- Lentils
- Lima beans
- Macadamia nut butter
- Macadamia nuts
- Millet
- Monkey nuts
- Mung beans
- Navy beans
- Nutmeg
- Oak nuts
- Olive pits
- Peanut butter
- Peanuts
- Peanuts in the shell
- Peas
- Pecans
- Pili nuts
- Pine nuts
- Pinto beans
- Pistachio butter
- Pistachios
- Poppy seeds
- Pumpkin seeds
- Quinoa
- Red beans
- Sesame seeds
- Sorghum
- Soy nuts
- Soybeans
- Split peas
- Sunflower seed butter
- Sunflower seeds
- Tahini
- Teff
- Tigernuts
- Walnuts
- Watermelon seeds
- White beans

- Almond milk
- Aloe vera juice
- Apple cider
- Apple juice
- Apricot nectar
- Beet juice
- Blackberry juice
- Blackberry tea
- Blueberry juice
- Blueberry slushie
- Blueberry
- Buttermilk
- Carrot juice
- Cashew milk
- Cherry juice
- Cherry slushie
- Cherry sorbet
- Club soda
- Coconut milk
- Coconut water
- Coffee (regular, decaf)
- Cola (check the label)
- Cold brew coffee
- Cow milk
- Cranberry juice
- Eggnog (check the label)
- Flax milk
- Fruit-infused water
- Ginger ale (check the label)
- Goat milk
- Grape juice
- Grape juice
- Grape slushie
- Grapefruit juice
- Grapefruit slushie
- Guava juice
- Hazelnut milk
- Hemp milk
- Horchata (check the label)
- Hot chocolate (check the label)
- Iced tea
- Kiwi-strawberry smoothie
- Kombucha
- Lemon sorbet
- Lemon tea
- Lemon-lime slushie
- Lemon-lime soda (check the label)
- Lemon-lime sports drinks (check the label)
- Lemonade
- Lemonade tea
- Lime sorbet
- Limeade
- Mango juice
- Mango nectar
- Mango sorbet
- Mango-pineapple smoothie
- Mineral water
- Oat milk (check the label)
- Orange juice
- Orange slushie
- Orange sorbet
- Orangeade
- Papaya juice
- Passionfruit juice
- Peach nectar
- Peach slushie
- Peach smoothie
- Peach sorbet
- Peach tea
- Peach-passionfruit tea
- Pear cider
- Pineapple juice
- Pineapple slushie
- Pineapple sorbet
- Pineapple-coconut juice
- Pineapple-coconut water
- Pineapple-orange juice
- Pomegranate juice
- Prune juice
- Quinoa milk
- Raspberry juice
- Raspberry slushie
- Raspberry sorbet
- Raspberry tea
- Raspberry-lemon tea
- Raspberry-mango smoothie
- Rice milk
- Root beer (check the label)
- Seltzer water
- Soy milk
- Sparkling water
- Strawberry juice
- Strawberry sorbet
- Strawberry-banana smoothie
- Strawberry-banana-peach smoothie
- Tea (herbal, black, green, white, etc.)
- Tomato juice
- Tonic water
- Water
- Watermelon slushie

- Ardrahan
- Asiago
- Bel Paese
- Blue cheese (check label to confirm)
- Brie
- Brunost
- Burrata
- Cabot Clothbound Cheddar
- Cabra al Vino
- Caciocavallo
- Caciotta
- Camembert
- Cantal
- Caprino
- Chaumes
- Cheddar
- Chèvre (goat cheese)
- Colby
- Comté
- Cotija
- Cottage cheese
- Cream cheese
- Crescenza
- Danish Blue
- Edam
- Emmental
- Etorki
- Feta
- Fontal
- Fontina
- Fourme d'Ambert
- Fourme de Montbrison
- Gjetost
- Gloucester
- Goat cheese (chevre)
- Gorgonzola (check label to confirm)
- Gouda
- Grana Padano
- Grès des Vosges
- Halloumi
- Havarti
- Herve
- Idiazabal
- Jarlsberg
- La Tur
- Lancashire
- Langres
- Le Fleuron
- Leerdammer
- Leerdammer
- Limburger
- Livarot
- Mahón
- Mahón-Menorca
- Manchego
- Manchego Curado
- Maroilles
- Mimolette
- Montasio
- Monterey Jack
- Morbier
- Mozzarella
- Muenster
- Munster-Géromé
- Oaxaca
- Ossau-Iraty
- Parmesan
- Pecorino
- Pecorino Calabrese
- Pecorino Crotonese
- Pecorino Moliterno
- Pecorino Romano
- Pecorino Sardo
- Pecorino Toscano
- Pepper Jack
- Piave
- Picón Bejes-Tresviso
- Port Salut
- Provolone
- Queso blanco
- Queso de Cabra
- Queso de Tetilla
- Queso fresco
- Raclette
- Raclette de Savoie
- Raschera
- Reblochon
- Red Leicester
- Ricotta
- Robiola
- Romano
- Roncal
- Roquefort (check label to confirm)
- Saint Agur
- Saint André
- Saint-Nectaire
- Sardo
- Selles-sur-Cher
- Serpa
- Serra da Estrela
- Shropshire Blue
- Swiss
- Taleggio
- Tête de Moine
- Toma Piemontese
- Tomme Crayeuse
- Tomme de Savoie
- Truffle cheese
- Tunworth
- Tybo
- Ubriaco
- Valdeón
- Valencay
- Vignotte

- Alfredo sauce
- Apple sauce
- Apricot halves
- Artichokes
- Asparagus
- Baked beans (check label to confirm)
- Balsamic vinaigrette
- BBQ sauce
- Beef broth
- Beef chili
- Beef ravioli
- Beef stew
- Beets
- Black beans
- Blue cheese dressing
- Butternut squash puree
- Caesar dressing
- Cannellini beans
- Capers
- Carrots
- Chicken and dumplings
- Chicken and rice soup
- Chicken broth
- Chicken noodle soup (check label to confirm)
- Chicken stew
- Chickpeas (garbanzo beans)
- Clams
- Cocktail sauce
- Coconut milk
- Coconut water
- Corn
- Corned beef hash
- Crab meat
- Cream of celery soup
- Cream of chicken soup
- Cream of mushroom soup
- Creamed corn
- Creamed spinach
- Diced tomatoes with green chilies
- Enchilada sauce
- Fruit cocktail
- Green beans
- Green chilies
- Hot sauce
- Italian dressing
- Ketchup
- Kidney beans
- Lentil soup
- Lima beans
- Lobster
- Mandarin orange segments
- Mandarin oranges
- Mango slices
- Marinara sauce
- Mayonnaise
- Minestrone soup
- Mushrooms
- Mustard
- Olives
- Orange juice
- Oysters
- Peach slices
- Peaches and cream corn
- Pear halves
- Pear sauce
- Peas
- Pesto sauce
- Pickles
- Pineapple chunks
- Pineapple juice
- Pineapple slices
- Pinto beans
- Pumpkin puree
- Ranch dressing
- Roasted red peppers
- Salmon
- Salsa
- Sardines
- Sauerkraut
- Shrimp
- Sloppy Joe sauce
- Soy sauce (check label to confirm)
- Spaghetti sauce
- Split pea soup
- Sweet potato puree
- Taco sauce
- Tartar sauce
- Teriyaki sauce
- Tomato juice
- Tomato paste
- Tomato sauce
- Tomato soup
- Tomatoes
- Tuna
- Turkey chili
- Vegetable broth
- Vegetable juice
- Vegetable soup
- Worcestershire sauce

Milton Keynes UK
Ingram Content Group UK Ltd.
UKHW021628090624
443713UK00018B/577

9 781399 962568